CARB CYCLING
FOR VEGANS

A Beginner's Step-by-Step Guide With Recipes and a Meal Plan

mindplusfood

FREE BONUS

Thank you for your purchase. Subscribe to mindplusfood.com for a free 41-Page holistic health and weight loss cheat sheet and exclusive wellness content

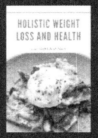

HOLISTIC WEIGHT
LOSS AND HEALTH

Disclaimer

By reading this disclaimer, you are accepting the terms of the disclaimer in full. If you disagree with this disclaimer, please do not read the guide. The content in this guide is provided for informational and educational purposes only.

This guide is not intended to be a substitute for the original work of this diet plan. At most, this guide is intended to be a beginner's supplement to the original work for this diet plan and never act as a direct substitute. This guide is an overview, review, and commentary on the facts of that diet plan.

All product names, diet plans, or names used in this guide are for identification purposes only and are the property of their respective owners. The use of these names does not imply endorsement. All other trademarks cited herein are the property of their respective owners.

None of the information in this guide should be accepted as independent medical or other professional advice.

The information in the guide has been compiled from various sources that are deemed reliable. It has been analyzed and summarized to the best of the Author's ability, knowledge, and belief. However, the Author cannot guarantee the accuracy and thus should not be held liable for any errors.

You acknowledge and agree that the Author of this guide will not be held liable for any damages, costs, expenses, resulting from the application of the information in this guide, whether directly or indirectly. You acknowledge and agree that you assume all risk and responsibility for any action you undertake in response to the information in this guide.

You acknowledge and agree that by continuing to read this guide, you will (where applicable, appropriate, or necessary) consult a qualified medical professional on this information. The information in this guide is not intended to be any sort of medical advice and should not be used in lieu of any medical advice by a licensed and qualified medical professional.

Always seek the advice of your physician or another qualified health provider with any issues or questions you might have regarding any sort of medical condition. Do not ever disregard any qualified professional medical advice or delay seeking that advice because of anything you have read in this guide.

TABLE OF CONTENTS

INTRODUCTION

Dieting is one of the most practiced lifestyles we have today. There are numerous reasons why people opt for a diet, either to lose weight, improve performance, or simply to maintain a healthy body. If you're one of those people who aim for such, then keep reading.

One of the important aspects of dieting involves being aware of the macronutrients in our food. These macronutrients are Fats, Cholesterol, Protein, Amino Acids, Fiber, and Carbohydrates.[1] Often, weight-loss diets are geared towards less carb intake and more protein intake. Why is that so?

Carbs are mostly found in sweet foods because it is made of sugar or starch. The body takes this starch and forms it into glucose, which is a primary source of energy for our body. Carbs can be classified as healthy and unhealthy. Healthy carbs can be found in fruits and vegetables, beans, and whole grains which aid in delivering nutrients. Unhealthy carbs, on the other hand, can be found in sodas, processed foods, and white bread. Often, these foods cause weight gain and the excessive intake of these carbs may lead to serious diseases like diabetes. [2]

Research has shown that less carb intake results in natural weight loss. It helps in decreasing your appetite and some people feel fuller and more satisfied with less carb intake.[3] However, eating very little amounts of carbohydrates will not allow your body to function properly due to a lack of sugar. Hypoglycemia, or low blood sugar, may happen. Your body will also undergo ketosis or burning fat for energy. [4]

Therefore, eating the right amount of carbs is very important in maintaining a healthy body. One way to do this is through carb cycling.

In this guide, we will show you:

- What carb cycling is
- How carb cycling is done for vegans
- The Advantages and disadvantages of carb cycling for vegans
- A brief example of a carb cycling plan for vegans.
- Healthy vegan recipes when going through carb cycling

CHAPTER I: WHAT EXACTLY IS CARB CYCLING?

Franco Carlotto, a 6-time Mr. World Fitness Champion created Carb Cycle out of the will to become a World Champion. Carb cycling is a form of diet that involves planned alternations of carb intake. It allows you to build muscles without gaining too much fat.

How Do You Start Carb Cycling?
Carb cycling is an effective diet when it's done properly. You can start it off by making meal plans, listing the foods to take during high, moderate, or low carbohydrates days. Second, think about the number of meals that you'd take a day. And lastly, monitor your diet routine and record its effects weekly to know if there's a change in your body.
There are different variations to carb cycling; it depends on what's best for your body and your ultimate goals.

It can be in the form of a 7-day meal plan where you take high-carbs and low-carbs alternately. This style is good for women who want to do carb cycling.

Other than that, you can try a longer period of the high and low-carb cycle. Depend it on your planned physical activities for the day.

- When you're in training or on heavy workout days, take

high-carb foods. With this, your body will use carbohydrates as energy fuel during workouts so your body won't experience fatigue.

- When you're at rest, start taking low-carbs to burn some fats. When your body doesn't have enough carbs to support your activities, it converts the stored fats into energy.

You can also try longer low-carb intake, then short periods of refeeding. After a long duration of a strict diet, reward yourself by having some refeeds or high-carb intake. Then go back to strict diet protocols to burn the fats that you stored during refeeding.

Carb cycling meal plan can change if your body is uncomfortable with the previous one or if it doesn't seem to help in achieving your goal.

Benefits from Carb Cycling

- **Weight and Fat Loss**

Carb cycling promotes calories deficit which will result in weight loss.

- **Muscle Gain**

If you're an athlete or a fan of extreme workouts, carb cycling is a good way to develop your muscles. Muscle-building workouts require great power, you can get enough energy to do this when you take high-carbs.

- **Others:**
  ❖ Low-carbohydrates intake improves insulin sensitivity and cholesterol levels. It also helps in enhancing the body's metabolism.
  ❖ High-carbohydrates intake or also knows as "refeed" which we did after a long period of the low-carb day helps in enhancing some hormones like thyroid hormones, testosterone, and leptin.

Is Carb Cycling safe?

Carb cycling is safe as long as you follow the diet protocols. However, if you take moderate-carbs and do excessive work, you might experience unusual fatigue. Engaging in low-carbohydrates intake while under the workout period may cause stress, fatigue and may also lead to serious illness because of a lack of energy fuel.

Women are more likely prone to fat tissues than men, this makes their diet quite stricter that they often choose a diet that sticks with carbohydrates starvation. That makes carb cycling the perfect dietary strategy for women, it allows them to gain muscles and lose fats without experiencing too much food restriction at all.

CHAPTER 2: WHAT IS CARB CYCLING FOR VEGANS?

Yes, vegans can carb cycle too, but it will be harder than non-vegans because of the limited alternatives that you can have.

In making your carb cycle plan, it is important to keep the other macronutrients in mind, mainly Carbohydrates, protein, and fat.

Carbohydrates

In this diet plan, Carbohydrates will be the main regulatory macronutrient you need to keep an eye on. There are days where you will have to eat high carb foods and low carb foods. A low carb day would mean that you would have to eat foods heavy on fat and vice versa. When choosing a carbohydrate source that you want to eat, it is best to avoid processed foods as they may have extra ingredients that would hinder your goals. Some of the foods that are rich in carbohydrates are: [5]

- Oats
- Potatoes
- Quinoa
- Rice and other rice products such as rice cakes
- Sweet Potatoes

For Low Carb days, the best foods to take are: [6] [7] [8]

- Blackberries
- Blueberries

- Broccoli
- Brussels Sprouts
- Cauliflower
- Dark chocolate
- Hemp seeds
- Lemon Juice
- MCT Oil
- Mushrooms
- Peppers
- Raspberries
- Sesame seeds
- Spinach
- Strawberries
- Vegetables
- Zucchini

For High Carb days, the best foods to take are:[9] [10]

- Quinoa
- Oats
- Buckwheat
- Bananas
- Sweet Potatoes
- Beetroots
- Oranges
- Grapefruit
- Apples
- Kidney Beans
- Chickpeas
- Rice
- Millet
- Spelt
- Whole grain pasta
- Bread
- Parsnips
- Pumpkin
- Squash

Protein

Protein is important in balancing out the lost carbs. It helps in making your muscles lean and strong. It also helps in making you feel fuller so the risks of overeating and unnecessary eating can be reduced. Often, protein is acquired in meat and fish products, but there are also a wide array of vegan foods that contain protein. Some of them are: [11] [12] [13]

- Almonds
- Amaranth
- Ancient grains like barley, einkorn, spelt, farro, and teff
- Beans like Lupini beans, pinto beans, and black beans
- Bread made from Sprouted Grains like Ezekiel Bread.
- Chia Seeds
- Chickpeas
- Edamame
- Green Peas
- Hempseed
- Hummus
- Lentils
- Natural Peanut butter
- Nut butter
- Nutritional yeast or vegan cheese
- Nuts
- Oatmeal
- Oats
- Plant-based Protein Powder
- Quinoa
- Seitan (A gluten food product that is used to make mock meat, therefore it is not ideal for people who are gluten sensitive)
- Soybeans (Fermented soybeans are the best option, avoid soy products that are processed since they might have ingredients that will make your diet harder.)
- Spirulina
- Sunflower seed butter

- Tahini
- Tempeh
- Tofu
- Wild Rice

Fats

Fats are essential in this diet because other than carbohydrates, the body will take fats as a source of energy as well. This is why taking in large amounts of fat on low carb days and small amounts of fat on high carb days makes the body balanced enough. Here is a list of foods rich in fat: [14] [15] [16]

- Almonds
- Avocado
- Cacao Nibs
- Coconut products like coconut milk, coconut oil, and coconut butter
- Ground Flaxseed
- Hemp seeds
- Macadamia nuts
- Nuts
- Olive Oil
- Olives
- Pumpkin Seeds
- Sesame Oil
- Shredded Coconut
- Sunflower seeds
- Walnuts

Recipes for meals that you can make

Low Carb Vegan Recipe Ideas
1. Roasted Veggies
Ingredients:
- ½ pounds of turnips
- ½ pounds of carrots
- ½ pounds of parsnips

- 2 peeled shallots (medium-sized)
- ¼ teaspoon of ground black pepper
- 2 tablespoon further of virgin coconut oil
- 6 cloves of garlic (with skin)
- ¾ teaspoon of kosher salt
- 2 tbsp of contemporary rosemary needles

Directions:

1. Cut vegetables into bite-sized items first
2. Set the kitchen appliance to 400°F.
3. Combine all the ingredients in a baking dish.
4. Roast the vegetables for twenty-five minutes
5. Toss and roast once more for twenty- twenty-five minutes.
6. Serve it hot.

2. Spinach and Watercress Salad

Ingredients

- 1 cup watercress, washed and stems removed
- 3 cups baby spinach, washed and stems removed
- 1 medium sliced avocado
- ½ cup Parmesan cheese, shredded
- ¼ cup avocado oil
- 1/8 cup lemon juice
- Salt and Pepper to taste
- 1 tbsp. Mediterranean seasoning (optional)

Instructions

1. Pat dry the spinach and watercress.
2. On a large serving plate, combine the leaves of the watercress and the spinach.
3. Cut the avocado in half then remove the pit. Peel the skin off from each side.
4. Slice the avocadoes into thin strips. Set it aside.
5. Prepare the dressing by combining avocado oil, lemon juice, and Mediterranean seasoning
6. Arrange the avocado strips on top of the watercress and

spinach. Top with shredded cheese and season with salt and pepper.
7. Drizzle with the dressing

3. Thai Salad with Coconut Curry Sauce

Ingredients
- For the dressing
- 1 can low-fat coconut milk
- 1/4 cup creamy peanut butter
- 1 tablespoon yellow curry powder
- 1 clove garlic
- juice of a lime
- 1-2 teaspoons sriracha
- 1 teaspoon kosher salt (or to taste)
- For the salad
- 3 cups chopped kale
- 2 cups chopped napa cabbage
- 1 red bell pepper (chopped)
- 1 cup shredded carrots
- 1 cup chopped mango
- 1/2 cup chopped peanuts
- 1/2 cup chopped cilantro

Instructions
1. Place all of the dressing ingredients in a blender and blend on high speed until very smooth. Place the dressing in a saucepan, bring to a boil then simmer until reduced and thickened, about 10 minutes.
2. Place the remaining ingredients into a large bowl, toss with the dressing and serve immediately.

High Carb Vegan Recipe Ideas

1. Vegan Corn and Potato Chowder

Ingredients
- 1 large sweet yellow onion – peeled and finely chopped
- 2 quarts of low-sodium vegetable broth

- 1/4 cup of white wine
- 3 cups of frozen yellow corn
- 3 medium potatoes – peeled and cubed
- 2 teaspoons of smoked paprika
- 1 teaspoon of ground white pepper
- 3 teaspoons of liquid smoke
- 1 and 1/2 teaspoons of finely ground sea salt
- 1 pinch of cayenne pepper

Instructions

1. In a large soup pot heat the three tablespoons of vegetable broth on medium-high heat. When the broth is hot add the onions and stir well.
2. Stir the onions occasionally. When they are slightly caramelized add the wine or vegetable broth and deglaze the pan)
3. Once the pot is deglazed add the remaining vegetable broth, corn, and potatoes. Stir to combine and bring to a boil. Reduce the heat to a low simmer and add the paprika, pepper, liquid smoke, salt, and cayenne pepper. Stir well.
4. Cook for approximately thirty minutes or until the potatoes are easily pierced with a fork.
5. Remove two cups of the soup from the pot and place in a small bowl. Set aside.
6. Use a blender to blend the remaining soup in the pot.

2. Vegan Mac and Cheese

INGREDIENTS

- 2 cups of water
- 1 sweet potato, peeled and chopped
- 8 baby carrots
- 1 zucchini, peeled and chopped
- 1/2 of a sweet onion, chopped
- 12 oz. of pasta
- CHEESE SAUCE
- boiled vegetables
- remaining water from the pot
- 1/2–3/4 cup nutritional yeast
- 1 tablespoon dijon mustard
- 1 clove garlic, minced
- 1 teaspoon salt, or to taste
- 3/4 teaspoon turmeric
- pepper, to taste
- dash of cayenne pepper (optional)

INSTRUCTIONS

1. In a small pot, bring 2 cups of water to a boil. Add in the sweet potato and boil for about 5 minutes. Add in the carrots, zucchini, and onion. Boil for another 5-8 minutes. Remove from heat.
2. In a separate pot, start boiling the water for the pasta. Cook 12 oz. of your favorite pasta. Drain and transfer pasta back to the pot.
3. Start making the cheese sauce. Spoon out the boiled vegetables and transfer them to a blender. Add in the remaining boiled water from that pot. Add in the rest of the ingredients for the cheese sauce.
4. Pour the cheese sauce over the pasta. Mix until well combined.

3. Spicy buddha bowl

Ingredients

- 1 cup Cooked Brown Rice
- 1 Sweet Potato, cut into large chunks
- 1 teaspoon Olive Oil
- Salt/Pepper
- 1 can Organic Chickpeas, drained
- 1 1/2 tablespoons Sriracha
- 2 teaspoons Maple Syrup
- 1/2 teaspoon Paprika
- 1/2 teaspoon Garlic Powder
- Salt/Pepper
- 1 cup chopped Red Cabbage
- 1 cup Baby Spinach
- 1 Avocado, sliced

Turmeric Tahini Dressing:
- 4 Tablespoons Tahini
- 4 Tablespoons Warm Water
- 1 teaspoon Maple Syrup
- 1/4 teaspoon Cayenne Pepper
- 1/2 teaspoon Turmeric
- 1/2 teaspoon Sriracha
- Salt to taste

Instructions

1. Preheat oven to 180 degrees Celsius. Coat sweet potato in 1 tsp oil and season with salt and pepper. Place on a baking tray and pop into the oven to roast for 35 minutes
2. Whilst sweet potato is cooking, prepare chickpeas.
3. In a bowl, combine chickpeas, sriracha, maple syrup, paprika, garlic powder, salt, and pepper. Mix to combine. Heat a saucepan and transfer chickpea mixture into a saucepan to cook for 5-10 minutes. Cook until chickpeas are slightly sticky
4. In a clean saucepan, wilt the spinach slightly and season. Transfer to a bowl and repeat

5. Place rice in the bottom of a bowl and then topping with the sweet potato, chickpeas, spinach, red cabbage, and avocado.

4. Vegan Tiramisu

Ingredients

CAKE

- 1 cup less 2 tbsps oat flour
- 2 1/2 tbsp corn starch
- 1/4 cup organic cane sugar
- 1/2 cup non-dairy milk
- 2 tbsps almond milk yogurt
- 1 tsp vanilla extract
- 2 tsp baking powder

PUDDING

- 8 pitted Medjool dates
- 2 cups non-dairy milk
- 2 tsp vanilla extract
- 3 tbsp corn starch
- 1 tbsp lemon juice
- 1/2 cup brewed coffee or Teeccino
- 1 tbsp of cacao powder
-

Instructions

FOR THE CAKE:

1. Preheat the oven to 350F.
2. Sift the oat flour, baking powder, and cornstarch into a mixing bowl.
3. Add the rest of the ingredients and whisk till smooth.
4. Pour a shallow layer of cake into the bottom of an 8×8" square pan lined with parchment paper.
5. Bake for 10-11 minutes until the center bounces back when touched.
6. Set aside to cool.

FOR THE PUDDING:

1. Blend all the ingredients on high till smooth.

2. Pour into a large heat-safe bowl.
3. Microwave on high for 1 minute. Whisk. Then micro-wave for another 1 minute on high until thickened.
4. Let it cool with a piece of plastic wrap on top so it doesn't form that weird layer.

TO ASSEMBLE:
1. Once everything is cool, cut the cake into cubes.
2. Briefly dip each cube into the coffee and layer them in the bottom of the glass.
3. Top with the pudding, a dusting of cacao powder

Advantages of Carb Cycling

Carb cycling has many benefits for the body, some of these benefits are:

1.   It helps in maintaining a healthy body weight

One of the best effects of carb cycling is helping a person lose weight or build muscle. Going on a maintained carb level for some time can help your body in regulating the energy it consumes and uses. When going through the low carb days, your body increases its insulin sensitivity that helps the body burn fat. High carb days, on the other hand, help your body recover from the lower carb intake, build muscle, as well as keeps your metabolism in check. This way, you are trying to lose weight without straining your body further and keeping its functions at bay. [17]

The diet is also said to have effects on getting body fat decreased. Eating less than the normal amount of carbohydrates will push your body into a state of ketosis. This is where the body begins to burn fat as a source of energy. It is like exercising without actually moving, you are burning fat because your body needs it as a source of energy now. [18]

2.   It can help in increasing your performance level

Carb cycling is done mostly by athletes and bodybuilders because of this advantage. By carb cycling, the body is trying to maintain healthy levels of glycogen. This glycogen works well in fueling our bodies when we do exercise, which in turn helps the muscles to grow. [19]

3.   It helps regulate your hormones

Through carb cycling, you are feeding your body what it needs only, not too much and not too little. This way, your food intake matches what the body only needs, which in turn makes hormone regulation better. The body also uses the carbohydrates in the right way, as a form of energy, which helps a person feel more energized, rejuvenated, and recovered better.

Hormones like ghrelin and leptin, or the hormones responsible for inducing and suppressing your appetite respectively,[20] are also being regulated under carb cycling on low carb days. On the other hand, high carb days also help in increasing your metabolism, which would make your body burn fat for energy at a faster scale, leading to weight loss. [21]

Disadvantages of Carb Cycling

While there are advantages of carb cycling, there are also disadvantages that may hinder your goals further or detriment your body. Therefore, it is important to be aware of these disadvantages before starting your carb cycling plan so that you can have the choice to proceed at your own risk or not. Some of the disadvantages of carb cycling are: [22]

1.   It may not be for everyone

As promising as it sounds, carb cycling may not be for everyone to try because there are certain parameters in your own body that you must be mindful of. While it is true that some athletes do improve their performance levels, there might be people who might lessen their stamina and strength because of the less carb intake. Some people might experience side effects from eating low carbs such as bloating, constipation, fatigue, irritability, sleep issues, and cravings. When these effects happen, it is important to listen to your body, stop the program immediately, and consult a doctor. Therefore, you really must be mindful of the way your body reacts to a certain diet before you partake in it fully.

Additionally, this diet is not suitable for people who have health issues such as heart diseases and diabetes. It is also not recommended for people diagnosed with eating disorders and pregnant and lactating women.

2.   Planning can be a hassle

As mentioned in the previous pointer, there are things in your body that you must be mindful of. Making a carb cycling plan might be taxing at first because the plan varies on the type of body that you have. No plan is the same as the other. You can try to make a basis of the plan presented in this guide, but ultimately you will have to create one of your own to ensure that the results can be maximized. A few things that are needed in creating a plan are:

- Age
- BMR or Basal Metabolic Rate
- Height
- How active you are (Light exercises, active, sedentary, etc.)
- Weight

3.   It needs strict planning and following

To maximize the effects of this plan, you need to follow it very carefully and make sure that you are eating according to your plan. One needs to be committed and patient to follow through with this diet, which can be hard for some people due to internal and external factors. You will also need a few tools that would help you calculate the macronutrients of the food you eat daily. It is quite a taxing thing to do, especially if you are a busy person.

Additionally, the program isn't sustainable. While some people can be committed to following it for a few months or so, one cannot do it for the rest of their lives. It is important that while you are on a diet, learn to make changes in your lifestyle, and not go back to it once the program is over. That way, long term effects can be seen.

CHAPTER 3: THE FIRST WEEK OF CARB CYCLING JOURNEY

Are you looking for a Carb Cycling diet plan? You can follow the weekly diet plan stated below. It was mentioned earlier that Carb Cycling is the process of alternating the intake of carbohydrates that's why it is necessary to have an organized plan.

In this guide, there will be a 3-week diet plan. Every week, there will be a minimal change in the carbohydrate intake. Furthermore, there will be a variation of physical activities, and carb and fat intake to maintain the balance.

There are 2 common methods of Carb Cycling. These are The High/Low Method and The High/Medium/Low Method. (source: www.jcdfitness.com)

- The High/Low Method – in this method, you will be undergoing a high carb day followed by a low carb day. A high carb day must cover at least 150 grams of carbohydrates intake while a low carb day must cover at most 100 grams of carbohydrates intake.
- The High/Medium/Low Method – in this method you will be undergoing a high carb day followed by a medium carb day and eventually a low carb day. High carb day must cover at least 150 grams of carbohydrates intake, medium carb day must cover between 100-150 grams of carbohydrates intake, while low carb day must cover at most 100 grams of carbohydrates intake.

Below is a diet plan table for week 1 (source:

www.healthline.com):

DAY	EXERCISE	CARB INTAKE	FAT INTAKE	AMOUNT OF CARBS
Monday	Weight Training	High Carb	Low Fat	200 g
Tuesday	Aerobic Exercise	Mod Carb	Mod Fat	100 g
Wednesday	Rest Day	Low Carb	High Fat	30 g
Thursday	Weight Training	High Carb	Low Fat	200 g
Friday	Weight Training	High Carb	Low Fat	200 g
Saturday	Rest Day	Low Carb	High Fat	30 g
Sunday	Rest Day	Low Carb	High Fat	30 g

Meanwhile, to make your diet plan more efficient, there are certain rules and guidelines you must consider. (source: www.mymetabolicmeals.com)
- ✓ In research, it was found that most people eating meals within an 8-10-hour gap burn more fatty acids, enhance insulin sensitivity, and reduce damaged cells. Thus, you must eat your meals within an exact gap.
- ✓ Protein can be an essential agent to create weight loss through soothing blood sugar and sustaining muscle mass. Thus, you must eat 20-40 grams of protein during your meals.
- ✓ Fiber supports the regulation of blood sugar, which is necessary to maintain regular body weight. Fiber can be gain by eating fruits and vegetables. Thus, you must eat vegetables during your meals.
- ✓ Prefer whole foods rather than powdered ones.
- ✓ To improve body composition, you need to intake around 3-6 grams of omega 3 fatty acids during your meal.

On the other hand, there are also certain things you need to avoid during your Carb Cycling diet. (source: www.mymetabolicmeals.com)
- ✓ Avoid flavored beverages and drinks. This kind of drink may be a hindrance to your progress during your diet properly. It is advisable to drink water and unsweetened teas rather than flavored ones.
- ✓ Follow your meal plan. Do not cheat on your plan to achieve progress within a couple of days or weeks.

✓ Avoid sauces. It is better to use spices rather than sauces like ketchup and dressings. This kind of seasonings contains a high amount of carbohydrates.

CHAPTER 4: SECOND WEEK OF CARB CYCLING JOURNEY

After your first week of the Carb Cycling journey, there are still two more weeks. For the second week, here is a diet plan you can follow.

DAY	EXERCISE	CARB INTAKE	FAT INTAKE	AMOUNT OF CARBS
Monday	Weight Training	High Carb	Low Fat	250 g
Tuesday	Aerobic Exercise	Mod Carb	Mod Fat	150 g
Wednesday	Rest Day	No Carb	High Fat	0 g
Thursday	Weight Training	High Carb	Low Fat	250 g
Friday	Aerobic Exercise	Mod Carb	Mod Fat	150 g
Saturday	Rest Day	Low Carb	High Fat	100 g
Sunday	Rest Day	No Carb	High Fat	0 g

As you're in two weeks of the carb cycling process, you should restrict your meal diet and keep the following tips mentioned before in the first week of carb cycling diet.

CHAPTER 5: THIRD WEEK OF CARB CYCLING JOURNEY

Here you go, the third week of your carb cycle journey, the table below is an example of a simultaneous carb cycling process for the third week. However, take note that you can repeat your routine for another week depending on what's in your guts.

After the first two weeks of the Carb Cycling journey, you can continue this for more weeks based on your body's need. For the second week, here is a diet plan you can follow.

DAY	EXERCISE	CARB INTAKE	FAT INTAKE	AMOUNT OF CARBS
Monday	Weight Training	High Carb	Low Fat	250 g
Tuesday	Aerobic Exercise	Mod Carb	Mod Fat	150 g
Wednesday	Weight Training	High Carb	High Fat	250 g
Thursday	Rest Day	No Carb	Low Fat	0 g
Friday	Aerobic Exercise	Mod Carb	Mod Fat	150 g
Saturday	Rest Day	Low Carb	High Fat	100 g
Sunday	Rest Day	Low Carb	High Fat	100 g

Still, the remarks for this week's routine are to follow the tips and guides in the first-week process can see the effectiveness of Carb Cycling.

If you want to enhance your carb cycling diet, try to keep track of your carb cycling calculator or try to put your routine in a PDF file, or any schedule organizer can track and keep your carb cycling in the process.

CONCLUSION

Thank you again for getting this guide.

If you found this guide helpful, please take the time to share your thoughts and post a review. It'd be greatly appreciated!

Thank you and good luck!

---

[1] "Macronutrients," US Department of Agriculture, National Agricultural Library, n.d., https://www.nal.usda.gov/fnic/macronutrients

[2] "The Nutrition Source," School of Public Health, Harvard T.H. Chan, September 18, 2012, https://www.hsph.harvard.edu/nutritionsource/carbohydrates/

[3] Kris Gunnars, "How Many Carbs Should you Eat per Day to Lose Weight?," *Healthline*, April 2, 2020, https://www.healthline.com/nutrition/how-many-carbs-per-day-to-lose-weight

[4] "Carbohydrate." GB Health Watch, n.d., https://www.gbhealthwatch.com/Nutrient-Carbohydrate-Symptoms.php

[5] "Carb Cycling For Vegetarians and Vegans," Hiitburn, n.d, https://hiitburn.com/carb-cycling-for-vegetarians-and-vegans/

[6] Joe Leech, "How to Eat Low-Carb as a Vegetarian or Vegan," *Healthline*, June 4, 2017, https://www.healthline.com/nutrition/low-carb-as-a-vegetarian

[7] Jillian Kubala, "Vegan Keto Diet Guide: Benefits, Foods, and Sample Menu," *Healthline*, October 2, 2018, https://www.healthline.com/nutrition/vegan-keto-diet

[8] Franziska Spritzler, "How to eat low carb as a vegan," *Diet Doctor*, November 6, 2020, https://www.dietdoctor.com/low-carb/vegan

[9] Adda Bjarnadottir, "12 High-Carb Foods That are Actually Super Healthy," *Healthline*, September 11, 2018, https://www.healthline.com/nutrition/12-healthy-high-carb-foods

[10] Alena Schowalter, "High Carb Low Fat Vegan Diet: All you Need to know," *Nutriciously*, June 19, 2016, https://nutriciously.com/high-carb-low-fat-vegan-diet/

[11] Alina Petre, "the 17 Best Protein Sources for Vegans and Vegetarians," *Healthline*, August 16, 2016, https://www.healthline.com/nutrition/protein-for-vegans-vegetarians

[12] Franziska Spritzler, "How to eat low carb as a vegan,"

[13] "Carb Cycling For Vegetarians and Vegans,"

[14] Franziska Spritzler, "How to eat low carb as a vegan,"

[15] Sarah-Jane Bedwell et al., "21 healthy high-fat foods to keep you full and satisfied," *Self*, September 30, 2020, https://www.self.com/story/9-high-fat-foods-actually-good-for-you

[16] Jonathan Engels, " The 5 Cleanest Sources of Plant-Based Fats," *One Green Planet*, March 2020, https://www.onegreenplanet.org/vegan-food/the-5-cleanest-sources-of-plant-based-fats/

[17] Alexandre Valente, "Carb cycling For Vegans: The Definitive Guide", *Vegan Foundry*, December 4, 2019, https://veganfoundry.com/carb-cycling-for-vegans-the-definitive-guide/

[18] "Carb cycling for vegans," Let's Eat Smart, May 21, 2019, https://www.letseatsmart.com/carb-cycling-for-vegans/

[19] "What is carb cycling? And is it safe for vegans??," Vegans Lounge, last modified February 5, 2019, https://veganslounge.com/fitness-health/what-is-carb-cycl-and-safe-for-vegans/

[20] Elaine Magee, "Your 'Hunger Hormones'," *Nourish by WebMD*, February 18, 2005, https://www.webmd.com/diet/features/your-hunger-hormones#

[21] Chelsea Debret, "Balancing Hormones with Plant-Based Carb Cycling", *One Green Planet*, 2019, https://www.onegreenplanet.org/natural-health/balancing-hormones-plant-based-carb-cycling/

[22] Darla Leal, "Is Carb Cycling an Effective Eating Strategy?," *Very Well Fit*, September 21, 2020, https://www.verywellfit.com/is-carb-cycling-an-effective-dietary-approach-4175794

Printed in Great Britain
by Amazon

84084761R00020